PREDIABETES

FOOD LIST

Copyright © 2023 by Sarah Thompson

All rights reserved

This copyrights page explains the legal rights and protections related to the content of this nonfiction book for readers and users. You understand that you have the right to access or use this book in any way, including reading, downloading, or sharing. Ownership and Intellectual Property Rights: The content, graphics, and other elements in this nonfiction book are all covered by copyright and other intellectual property laws. Sarah Thompson is the only owner of the content. Any unauthorized use or reproduction of this book's content may be illegal and give rise to legal action. For reading and using this book for personal, non-commercial uses only, you have been granted a constrained, non-exclusive, and non-transferable permission. You are prohibited from altering, distributing or Without Sarah Thompson's prior written approval, you may not distribute, communicate, display, perform, reproduce, publish, license, create derivative works from, transfer, or sell any portion of the book.

INTRODUCTION

The Prediabetes Food List

In a world where dietary choices play an increasingly pivotal role in our well-being, "The Prediabetes Food List" emerges as an indispensable guide for individuals seeking to take control of their health journey. Authored with meticulous research and expert insight, this book is a comprehensive resource tailored to those on the cusp of a critical juncture: prediabetes.

With the global prevalence of prediabetes steadily on the rise, understanding the nuances of dietary intervention is paramount. This book transcends the traditional notion of a mere list, as it serves as a beacon of empowerment, enlightenment, and sustainable change. Immerse yourself in a wealth of knowledge that not only outlines which foods to embrace and avoid, but delves deeper into the scientific underpinnings, meal planning strategies, and lifestyle adjustments that can significantly impact your prediabetic journey.

Whether you're a health-conscious individual proactively seeking to thwart the onset of diabetes or someone recently diagnosed with prediabetes, this guide extends a helping hand. It transforms the concept of a simple food list into a transformative tool for cultivating mindful eating habits, making informed choices, and paving a path towards a healthier future. "The Prediabetes Food List" is more than a book; it's a vital companion on your quest to reclaim your well-being and embrace a life of vitality.

TABLE OF CONTENT

Baked cod with quinoa and sautéed spinach

Chicken and vegetable curry with cauliflower rice

Quinoa-stuffed bell peppers with lean ground turkey or tofu

Spinach and feta omelet with whole wheat toast

Baked tofu with roasted sweet potatoes and steamed green beans

Black bean and vegetable enchiladas with a side of salsa and brown rice

Grilled shrimp skewers with a side salad and whole grain couscous

Veggie and bean burrito bowl with brown rice and salsa.

GRILLED CHICKEN BREAST WITH STEAMED VEGETABLES

Grilled chicken breast with steamed vegetables is a nutritious and delicious meal option that can benefit individuals with prediabetes. This dish offers a balanced combination of lean protein and low-carbohydrate vegetables, which helps regulate blood sugar levels and promotes overall health.

The grilled chicken breast provides a lean source of protein that helps maintain muscle mass and keeps you feeling satisfied after a meal. It is low in saturated fat and contains essential amino acids that assist in supporting a healthy weight and managing blood sugar. Additionally, chicken breast is a rich source of vitamins and minerals, including B vitamins and selenium, which are important for energy production and immune function.

Steamed vegetables, on the other hand, offer a wide array of essential nutrients while being low in carbohydrates and calories. Vegetables such as broccoli, carrots, and green beans are packed with fiber, vitamins, and antioxidants, which are beneficial for managing blood sugar levels and promoting heart health. Steaming the vegetables helps retain their nutrients, resulting in a flavorful and wholesome addition to the meal.

To prepare this dish, start by marinating the chicken breast in a mixture of olive oil, lemon juice, garlic, and herbs for added flavor. Grilled the chicken until it is cooked through and juicy. Meanwhile, steam the vegetables until they are tender yet slightly crisp. Season them with a sprinkle of salt, pepper, and any additional herbs or spices. Serve the grilled chicken breast alongside the steamed vegetables for a well-rounded and diabetes-friendly meal option.

BAKED SALMON WITH QUINOA AND ROASTED BRUSSELS SPROUTS

"Baked salmon with quinoa and roasted Brussels sprouts" is a delicious and wholesome meal that offers numerous benefits for individuals with prediabetes. The star of this dish, salmon, is an excellent source of high-quality protein and omega-3 fatty acids, which have been shown to promote heart health and reduce inflammation, both important factors in managing prediabetes. Quinoa, a gluten-free grain, provides complex carbohydrates and fiber, aiding in blood sugar regulation and helping to control post-meal glucose levels. Additionally, quinoa contains essential minerals such as magnesium and potassium, which support the body's overall metabolic functions. Roasted Brussels sprouts, on the other hand, offer plenty of dietary fiber, vitamins, and antioxidants, contributing to better blood sugar control and reducing the risk of heart disease. The preparation of this dish involves marinating the salmon fillets in a mixture of lemon juice, garlic, and herbs before baking until it reaches a flaky texture. Simultaneously, Brussels sprouts are seasoned with olive oil, salt, and pepper, then roasted to a crispy perfection. Finally, fluffy quinoa is prepared separately and served as a base for the baked salmon and roasted Brussels sprouts, creating a well-balanced and flavorful combination. This wholesome meal not only promotes stable blood sugar levels but also satisfies taste buds, making it an excellent choice for individuals with prediabetes.

TURKEY CHILI WITH MIXED BEANS AND VEGETABLES

Turkey chili with mixed beans and vegetables is a delicious and nutritious dish that is suitable for individuals with prediabetes. This hearty meal not only satisfies one's taste buds but also offers numerous health benefits. Packed with protein from lean turkey, fiber from mixed beans, and an array of vitamins and minerals from a variety of vegetables, this chili is an ideal choice for maintaining stable blood sugar levels.

Turkey, as a lean source of protein, is crucial for prediabetic individuals as it provides essential amino acids without adding excessive saturated fats. The mixed beans, such as kidney beans, black beans, and chickpeas, are loaded with fiber that aids in slow digestion and helps prevent sudden spikes in blood sugar levels. Additionally, the vegetable medley, which can include ingredients like bell peppers, onions, tomatoes, zucchini, carrots, and corn, adds both flavor and essential nutrients. These vegetables are rich in vitamins A and C, antioxidants, and dietary fiber that contribute to better overall health and blood sugar control.

The preparation of turkey chili with mixed beans

and vegetables is relatively simple. Start by browning ground turkey in a large pot or skillet, using non-stick cooking spray to minimize added fats. Once the turkey is cooked, add in finely chopped onions, bell peppers, and minced garlic. Sauté until the vegetables become tender and fragrant. Next, add in canned mixed beans, preferably rinsed thoroughly to reduce sodium content, along with canned diced tomatoes. For additional spice and flavor, incorporate chili powder, cumin, paprika, and a pinch of cayenne pepper. Allow the mixture to simmer over medium heat for approximately 20-30 minutes to allow the flavors to meld together.

The end result is a hearty and flavorful turkey chili, packed with a variety of vegetables and beans, perfect for individuals with prediabetes looking to improve their overall health and maintain stable blood sugar levels. This wholesome meal can be enjoyed on its own or served with a side of brown rice or whole-grain bread for added fiber and sustained energy. Regular consumption of this balanced dish can contribute to improved blood sugar management, weight control, and overall well-being.

GRILLED STEAK WITH A SIDE SALAD AND ROASTED SWEET POTATOES

Grilled steak with a side salad and roasted sweet potatoes is a delicious and nutritious meal that is suitable for individuals with prediabetes. This well-balanced dish offers numerous benefits for managing blood sugar levels and improving overall health.

Starting with the grilled steak, it provides a good source of protein, which helps stabilize blood sugar levels and promotes satiety. Protein takes longer to digest, preventing quick spikes in blood glucose levels. It also aids in building and repairing tissues, supporting muscle strength and growth. Opting for lean cuts of steak, such as sirloin or tenderloin, ensures a lower intake of saturated fat, reducing the risk of heart disease, a common concern for those with prediabetes.

Accompanying the steak, the side salad adds an array of vitamins, minerals, and fiber. Leafy greens like spinach, kale, or romaine lettuce are high in nutrients and low in calories, thus aiding weight management, another important aspect of prediabetes management. Fiber-rich vegetables, such as cucumbers, bell peppers, and tomatoes, contribute to better blood glucose control by slowing down the absorption of carbohydrates. Additionally, the salad can be topped with healthy fats like avocado or nuts, which aid in better nutrient absorption and improve insulin sensitivity.

To complete the meal, roasted sweet potatoes offer an excellent alternative to starchy sides like white rice or mashed potatoes. Sweet potatoes have a lower glycemic index, meaning they cause a slower rise in blood sugar levels compared to high-glycemic foods. They are also rich in fiber, vitamins A and C, potassium, and antioxidants, all of which contribute to improved blood sugar regulation and overall well-being.

Preparing this dish is relatively simple. Season the steak with desired spices and grill it to your preferred level of doneness. Meanwhile, toss together a variety of fresh vegetables and leafy greens to create a colorful and nutritious side salad. Finally, coat sweet potato chunks with a small amount of olive oil, sprinkle with seasoning, and roast them in the oven until tender and slightly caramelized.

In conclusion, grilled steak with a side salad and roasted sweet potatoes is an excellent choice for individuals with prediabetes. This meal offers numerous benefits, including blood sugar control, weight management, nutrient intake, and improved insulin sensitivity. By incorporating this dish into their diet, individuals with prediabetes can enjoy a delicious and nourishing meal while supporting their health goals.

LEMON GARLIC SHRIMP WITH WHOLE WHEAT PASTA AND STEAMED BROCCOLI

Lemon garlic shrimp with whole wheat pasta and steamed broccoli is a delicious and healthy meal option for individuals with prediabetes. This dish offers numerous benefits for managing blood sugar levels and promoting overall well-being.

Starting with the main ingredient, shrimp is an excellent source of lean protein. Protein is vital for those with prediabetes as it helps stabilize blood sugar levels and provides a steady release of energy. Shrimp is also low in saturated fat, making it a heart-healthy choice. Moreover, the lemon and garlic in this recipe add a burst of flavor without the need for excessive amounts of sodium or added sugars, making it suitable for prediabetic individuals.

Whole wheat pasta is a complex carbohydrate that takes longer to digest compared to refined grains. As a result, it causes a slower and more gradual rise in blood glucose levels. This feature is crucial in managing prediabetes since it helps prevent sudden spikes in blood sugar. Additionally, whole wheat pasta is rich in dietary fiber, which aids in digestion, promotes satiety, and helps regulate blood sugar levels.

The inclusion of steamed broccoli further enhances the nutritional value of this meal. Broccoli is packed with essential vitamins and minerals such as vitamin C, vitamin K, and folate. Additionally, it is low in calories and carbohydrates while providing a good amount of fiber. Fiber is particularly beneficial for those with prediabetes as it slows down the digestion and absorption of carbohydrates, helping to stabilize blood sugar levels.

The preparation of this dish is relatively simple. Start by sautéing the shrimp in a mixture of olive oil, minced garlic, and lemon juice. Once cooked, remove the shrimp and set them aside. In the same pan, add cooked whole wheat pasta, steamed broccoli florets, and a squeeze of lemon juice. Toss the ingredients together until well combined, and then add back the shrimp. Serve hot and garnish with freshly chopped parsley, grated lemon zest, and a sprinkle of black pepper.

Overall, lemon garlic shrimp with whole wheat pasta and steamed broccoli is a balanced and nutritious meal choice that offers numerous benefits for individuals with prediabetes. By incorporating lean protein, whole grains, and fiber-rich vegetables, this dish assists in the

management of blood sugar levels, promotes
satiety, and ensures a well-rounded and tasty meal
option.

GREEK SALAD WITH GRILLED CHICKEN OR SHRIMP

Greek salad with grilled chicken or shrimp is an excellent choice for individuals with prediabetes due to its low glycemic index and nutrient-rich ingredients. This flavorful and satisfying dish combines crisp and refreshing vegetables, such as cucumbers, tomatoes, and red onions, with tangy Kalamata olives, creamy feta cheese, and a light dressing of olive oil and lemon juice. The salad is then complemented by lean, protein-packed grilled chicken or shrimp, making it a well-balanced meal option for those looking to manage their blood sugar levels.

The primary benefit of Greek salad for individuals with prediabetes is its low glycemic index. The glycemic index (GI) is a measurement of how certain foods affect blood sugar levels. Foods with a high GI can cause a sharp increase in blood sugar levels, which can be problematic for individuals with prediabetes. However, Greek salad is predominantly made up of vegetables, which have a low GI. This means that the carbohydrates in the salad are digested and absorbed more slowly, resulting in a steady release of glucose into the bloodstream and preventing major spikes in blood sugar levels.

Additionally, Greek salad offers a wide array of essential nutrients. The various vegetables provide vitamins, minerals, and antioxidants that contribute to overall health and wellbeing. Cucumbers are hydrating and rich in vitamins C and K, while tomatoes are packed with lycopene, an antioxidant that has been associated with a reduced risk of certain chronic diseases. Furthermore, Kalamata olives are a source of heart-healthy monounsaturated fats, and feta cheese supplies calcium and protein. The addition of grilled chicken or shrimp adds lean protein, which is essential for supporting muscle health and promoting satiety.

Preparing Greek salad with grilled chicken or shrimp is relatively simple. Begin by grilling the chicken or shrimp until cooked through and slightly charred for extra flavor. While the protein is cooking, chop the cucumbers, tomatoes, and red onions into bite-sized pieces. Combine these vegetables with Kalamata olives and crumbled feta cheese in a large bowl. In a separate small bowl, whisk together olive oil, lemon juice, salt, and pepper to create the dressing. Pour the dressing over the salad mixture and toss gently to coat all the ingredients evenly. Finally, top the salad with the grilled chicken or shrimp, and it is ready to serve. This nutritious and delicious Mediterranean-inspired dish provides a satisfying meal while supporting blood sugar management for individuals with prediabetes.

VEGETABLE STIR-FRY WITH TOFU OR LEAN BEEF

Vegetable stir-fry with tofu or lean beef is a delicious and nutritious meal option that can be highly beneficial for individuals with prediabetes. Packed with an array of colorful vegetables and protein-rich tofu or lean beef, this dish provides a satisfying and balanced meal that can help stabilize blood sugar levels and support overall health.

The benefits of this dish lie in its low glycemic index, which means it causes a relatively slower and gradual increase in blood sugar levels compared to high glycemic index foods. The inclusion of a variety of vegetables, such as bell peppers, broccoli, carrots, and snow peas, ensures a good intake of essential vitamins, minerals, and dietary fiber. These nutrients help to enhance insulin sensitivity, improve blood sugar control, and lower the risk of developing chronic conditions associated with prediabetes, such as heart disease and obesity.

The preparation of vegetable stir-fry with tofu or lean beef is fairly simple and can be customized to personal preferences. Start by cutting the vegetables into bite-sized pieces and the tofu or lean beef into thin strips. In a heated non-stick pan or wok, add a small amount of heart-healthy oil, such as olive oil or sesame oil. Add garlic and ginger for added flavor and sauté for a minute. Then, add the tofu or lean beef and cook until browned. Next, toss in the vegetables and stir-fry until they become tender yet still slightly crisp. To enhance the flavors, you can season with low-sodium soy sauce, a sprinkle of sesame seeds, or a drizzle of honey. Serve it over a bed of cooked brown rice or whole grain noodles for a satisfying and balanced meal.

By incorporating vegetable stir-fry with tofu or lean beef into a prediabetic diet, individuals can enjoy a tasty meal that helps regulate blood sugar levels, maintain a healthy weight, and support overall well-being. Remember to consume in moderation and combine this dish with regular exercise and a well-rounded diet for optimal benefits.

BAKED CHICKEN WITH BROWN RICE AND ROASTED ASPARAGUS

Baked chicken with brown rice and roasted asparagus is a delicious and nutritious meal that can be particularly beneficial for individuals with prediabetes. This wholesome dish offers a combination of lean protein, whole grains, and fiber-rich vegetables, providing essential nutrients while helping to regulate blood sugar levels.

The tender and flavorful baked chicken serves as an excellent source of lean protein. Protein is essential for maintaining and repairing body tissues, and it also helps to keep you feeling full and satisfied for longer periods, preventing overeating or snacking on unhealthy options. Additionally, lean protein aids in stabilizing blood sugar levels by slowing down the release of glucose into the bloodstream. Opting for baked chicken rather than fried variations further reduces the intake of unhealthy fats and calories.

Brown rice, a whole grain, is a healthier alternative to white rice due to its higher fiber content. Fiber plays a significant role in managing prediabetes as it helps control blood sugar levels by slowing down the absorption of glucose. It also promotes digestive health and reduces the risk of heart disease. Brown rice is packed with vitamins, minerals, and antioxidants, contributing to improved overall health.

Roasted asparagus completes this meal with its numerous health benefits. Asparagus is a low-calorie vegetable rich in vitamins A, C, and K, as well as folate and potassium. These nutrients are essential for maintaining healthy blood pressure and supporting cardiovascular health. Asparagus also contains a unique antioxidant called glutathione, which aids in preventing cellular damage and reducing inflammation in the body. Furthermore, the fiber content in asparagus assists with proper digestion and blood sugar regulation.

To prepare this nutritious meal, start by marinating the chicken with herbs, spices, and a touch of olive oil for added flavor. Place the marinated chicken in the oven to bake until fully cooked and tender. Meanwhile, cook the brown rice according to package instructions, ensuring fluffy and perfectly cooked grains. Trim the asparagus, toss them in olive oil, salt, and pepper, and roast them in the oven until crisp and slightly caramelized. Serve the baked chicken over a bed of brown rice and alongside the roasted asparagus for a balanced, wholesome, and satisfying meal that supports healthy blood sugar management.

QUINOA SALAD WITH MIXED VEGETABLES AND GRILLED SHRIMP

Quinoa salad with mixed vegetables and grilled shrimp is a delicious and nutritious dish that is perfect for individuals with prediabetes. This recipe combines the health benefits of quinoa, an ancient grain, with an array of colorful vegetables and lean protein. Quinoa is a great choice for prediabetes as it has a low glycemic index, which means it does not cause a sharp rise in blood sugar levels after consuming it. It is also high in fiber, protein, and essential nutrients such as magnesium, zinc, and iron, all of which are important for maintaining optimal health.

The preparation of this salad is quite simple. Begin by cooking the quinoa according to the package instructions and let it cool. Meanwhile, prepare the mixed vegetables by chopping a variety of vibrant vegetables like bell peppers, cherry tomatoes, cucumbers, and red onions. These vegetables are rich in vitamins, minerals, and antioxidants that can help reduce the risk of chronic diseases associated with prediabetes. Once the quinoa has cooled, toss it together with the mixed vegetables in a large bowl.

For the grilled shrimp, marinate them in a mixture

of olive oil, garlic, lemon juice, and a pinch of salt and pepper for added flavor. Grill the shrimp for a few minutes on each side until they turn pink and opaque. Shrimp is a lean source of protein that contains omega-3 fatty acids, which have been shown to improve insulin sensitivity and reduce inflammation associated with prediabetes.

To assemble the salad, add the grilled shrimp on top of the quinoa and vegetable mixture. Drizzle a homemade dressing made from olive oil, lemon juice, minced garlic, and herbs like parsley and basil. This light and tangy dressing adds a refreshing taste to the salad without adding excessive calories or sugar.

By incorporating this quinoa salad with mixed vegetables and grilled shrimp into a prediabetic diet, individuals can enjoy a satisfying meal while keeping their blood sugar levels stable. The combination of quinoa, vegetables, and shrimp provides a balanced mix of essential nutrients, fiber, and protein that can help regulate blood sugar, promote weight management, and reduce the risk of complications associated with prediabetes.

LENTIL SOUP WITH A SIDE OF WHOLE GRAIN BREAD

Lentil soup with a side of whole grain bread is a wholesome and nourishing meal option for individuals with prediabetes. Lentils, a legume rich in protein and fiber, are the main ingredient in this soup, providing numerous health benefits. The low glycemic index of lentils helps regulate blood sugar levels, making them an excellent choice for prediabetic individuals. Additionally, lentils are packed with essential nutrients such as iron, magnesium, and folate, which play a crucial role in overall health and wellbeing.

The accompanying whole grain bread provides complex carbohydrates, which are beneficial in managing prediabetes. Unlike refined grains, whole grains are rich in fiber, offering a slow and steady release of glucose into the bloodstream, preventing blood sugar spikes. The fiber in whole grain bread also aids in digestion and helps maintain a healthy weight, which is crucial for prediabetic individuals. Moreover, whole grain bread is a good source of vitamins and minerals that support a balanced diet.

Preparing lentil soup with a side of whole grain bread is relatively simple. To begin, thoroughly rinse and drain the lentils before cooking. In a large pot, sauté onions, garlic, and other desired vegetables such as carrots and celery in a small amount of olive oil until they are tender. Add the lentils and vegetable broth to the pot, along with desired spices such as cumin, paprika, and thyme. Bring the mixture to a boil, then reduce the heat and let it simmer until the lentils are cooked and tender, usually around 25-30 minutes. Season with salt and pepper to taste.

Alongside the soup, whole grain bread can be toasted or served as is. To ensure the bread is truly whole grain, check the label for words like "whole wheat" or "whole grain" as the first ingredient. Whole grain bread can be enjoyed sliced and topped with a healthy spread such as hummus or avocado.

Incorporating lentil soup with a side of whole grain bread into a prediabetic diet not only offers a satisfying and flavorsome meal but also promotes stable blood sugar levels. The combination of protein, fiber, and complex carbohydrates in this meal helps maintain a balanced diet while supporting optimal health for individuals with prediabetes.

GRILLED VEGETABLE WRAP WITH HUMMUS AND AVOCADO

The Grilled vegetable wrap with hummus and avocado is a delicious and nutritious option for individuals with prediabetes. This wrap not only offers a burst of flavors but also provides numerous health benefits. The combination of grilled vegetables, hummus, and avocado ensures a filling and satisfying meal that helps to maintain stable blood sugar levels.

Grilled vegetables are low in calories and high in fiber, making them an ideal choice for those with prediabetes. These vegetables, such as bell peppers, zucchini, and eggplant, are packed with essential vitamins and minerals that support overall health. Grilling the vegetables enhances their natural flavors and adds a smoky taste, making them even more enjoyable.

Hummus, a popular Middle Eastern dip made from chickpeas, is a fantastic addition to this wrap. Chickpeas are high in fiber and have a low glycemic index, which means they release sugar into the bloodstream slowly, preventing spikes in blood sugar levels. Additionally, hummus is a good source of plant-based protein, making it an excellent substitute for high-glycemic ingredients like processed meats or cheese.

Avocado is another star ingredient in this recipe, known for its health-promoting properties. Rich in healthy fats, avocados can help improve insulin sensitivity and maintain a stable blood sugar level. They are also loaded with fiber and essential nutrients like potassium and folate, which contribute to heart health and overall well-being.

To prepare this delicious wrap, start by grilling the vegetables until they become tender and slightly charred. Then, spread a generous amount of hummus over a whole wheat or low-carb tortilla. Next, layer the grilled vegetables on top of the hummus and add slices of ripe avocado. You can also include some fresh spinach or other leafy greens for added nutritional value. Finally, roll up the tortilla tightly and secure it with a toothpick or wrap it in parchment paper for easy handling.

This Grilled vegetable wrap with hummus and avocado provides a balanced combination of vegetables, healthy fats, protein, and fiber, all of which contribute to stabilizing blood sugar levels and promoting overall health. By incorporating this delicious and nutritious wrap into their diet, individuals with prediabetes can enjoy a flavorful meal that supports their wellness goals.

TUNA SALAD ON WHOLE GRAIN BREAD WITH A SIDE OF RAW VEGGIES

Tuna salad on whole grain bread with a side of raw veggies is a delicious and nutritious meal option suitable for individuals with prediabetes. This meal offers various benefits, starting with the whole grain bread, which provides dietary fiber. Fiber aids in digestion, keeps blood sugar levels stabilized, and helps manage weight by promoting a feeling of fullness. Additionally, whole grain bread contains essential nutrients such as vitamins, minerals, and antioxidants.

The tuna salad is another key component of this meal that provides numerous health benefits. Tuna is a lean source of protein that is low in saturated fat and high in omega-3 fatty acids. These fatty acids have been linked to improving heart health, reducing inflammation, and enhancing insulin sensitivity. The protein content in tuna aids in blood sugar regulation, preventing spikes and crashes that can exacerbate prediabetes symptoms.

Accompanying the tuna salad, the raw veggies in this meal contribute additional vital nutrients and dietary fiber. Raw vegetables like carrots, cucumbers, and bell peppers are rich in vitamins, minerals, and antioxidants that support overall health and reduce the risk of chronic diseases associated with prediabetes. The natural fiber present in raw vegetables further assists in glucose control, as it slows down the absorption of sugar into the bloodstream.

To prepare this meal, start by making the tuna salad. Drain and flake canned tuna in water or brine, and mix it with Greek yogurt, diced celery, chopped red onion, lemon juice, and seasonings like black pepper or dill. Adjust the seasoning and consistency according to personal taste preferences. Next, lightly toast a slice of whole grain bread, preferably one with fewer added sugars. Spread the tuna salad evenly on the bread, allowing for a generous amount. For the side of raw veggies, wash and slice any desired crunchy vegetables. Carrot sticks, cucumber slices, and bell pepper strips are all great choices. Serve the tuna salad sandwich alongside the raw veggies and enjoy a satisfying and nutritious meal that supports blood sugar management and overall health. This delicious meal option combines the benefits of whole grain bread, lean protein from tuna, and nutrient-rich raw vegetables to create a balanced and diabetes-friendly plate.

BAKED COD WITH QUINOA AND SAUTÉED SPINACH

Baked cod with quinoa and sautéed spinach is a delicious and nutritious meal that is perfect for individuals with prediabetes. This wholesome dish offers numerous benefits for managing blood sugar levels and promoting overall health.

Cod, a lean and low-calorie fish, is an excellent source of high-quality protein. Including protein-rich foods in your diet can help regulate blood sugar levels and increase satiety, preventing hunger pangs and overeating. Additionally, cod is rich in omega-3 fatty acids, which have been shown to reduce inflammation and lower the risk of heart disease, a common complication in people with prediabetes.

Quinoa, a gluten-free whole grain, is packed with fiber, protein, and essential nutrients. The fiber content in quinoa slows down the digestion process, preventing rapid spikes in blood sugar levels. Furthermore, quinoa is considered a low glycemic index food, meaning it has a minimal impact on blood sugar levels. By incorporating quinoa into your meal, you can promote stable blood sugar control and reduce the risk of developing type 2 diabetes.

Sautéed spinach adds a vibrant and nutritious element to the dish. Spinach is a nutrient powerhouse, rich in vitamins A, C, and K, as well as minerals like iron and magnesium. It is also low in calories and carbohydrates, making it an excellent choice for people with prediabetes. The high fiber content in spinach can aid in maintaining healthy blood sugar levels and assist with weight management.

To prepare this delicious meal, start by seasoning the cod fillets with salt, pepper, and your choice of herbs or spices. Place the seasoned fish in a baking dish and bake it in the oven until it becomes tender and flaky. Meanwhile, cook the quinoa according to package instructions, using chicken or vegetable broth for added flavor. In a separate pan, heat olive oil and sauté the spinach until wilted. Finally, serve the baked cod on a bed of quinoa and top it with the sautéed spinach.

In conclusion, the baked cod with quinoa and sautéed spinach is not only a flavorful dish but also provides various benefits for individuals with prediabetes. From its protein-packed cod to the low glycemic index quinoa and fiber-rich spinach, this meal offers a balanced combination of nutrients that can help manage blood sugar levels, reduce inflammation, and support overall health.

CHICKEN AND VEGETABLE CURRY WITH CAULIFLOWER RICE

Chicken and vegetable curry with cauliflower rice is a delicious and healthy option for individuals with prediabetes. This flavorful dish offers a wide range of benefits, both in terms of taste and nutrition.

The chicken in this curry provides a lean source of protein, which is important for individuals with prediabetes. Protein helps to stabilize blood sugar levels and can prevent post-meal spikes that are often associated with this condition. Additionally, chicken is low in fat, making it a heart-healthy choice.

The vegetables included in this curry are not only packed with essential nutrients, but they also add a burst of color and flavor to the dish. Vegetables such as bell peppers, carrots, and spinach are rich in vitamins, minerals, and antioxidants, which can help protect against chronic diseases like diabetes. These vegetables are also low in calories and high in fiber, promoting satiety and aiding in weight management – a crucial aspect of prediabetes management.

One of the highlights of this dish is the cauliflower rice. It is a clever low-carb alternative to traditional rice that makes it suitable for individuals with prediabetes. Cauliflower is an excellent source of fiber, vitamins C and K, and antioxidants. Its mild flavor and rice-like texture make it a perfect accompaniment to the flavorsome curry.

Preparing this dish is simple and requires a few steps. Start by cooking the chicken until it is tender and cooked through. In a separate pan, sauté the vegetables with fragrant spices like turmeric, cumin, and coriander. Once softened, add the chicken and a can of diced tomatoes. Simmer the mixture until the flavors meld together. While the curry is simmering, use a food processor to pulse the cauliflower florets into rice-like grains. Steam or sauté the cauliflower rice until it reaches the desired tenderness, and season it with salt and pepper to taste. Serve the chicken and vegetable curry over the cauliflower rice, and garnish with fresh cilantro for added flavor and visual appeal.

Overall, this chicken and vegetable curry with cauliflower rice is a nutritious and flavorful option for individuals with prediabetes. It offers a balanced combination of lean protein, vegetables, and a low-carb base, making it an ideal choice for those striving to manage blood sugar levels effectively.

QUINOA-STUFFED BELL PEPPERS WITH LEAN GROUND TURKEY OR TOFU

Quinoa-stuffed bell peppers with lean ground turkey or tofu is a nutritious and delicious meal option for individuals with prediabetes. This recipe offers numerous benefits as it combines the goodness of quinoa, fiber-rich bell peppers, and a choice between lean ground turkey or tofu for added protein.

Quinoa is a highly nutritious grain that is rich in fiber, protein, vitamins, and minerals. It is a low-glycemic index food, meaning it has minimal impact on blood sugar levels. This is particularly beneficial for individuals with prediabetes as it helps regulate blood sugar levels and prevent spikes. Quinoa is also an excellent source of magnesium, which is essential for managing insulin sensitivity and preventing the development of type 2 diabetes.

Bell peppers, on the other hand, are packed with antioxidants, vitamins A and C, and fiber. They are low in calories and have a low glycemic index, making them suitable for individuals with prediabetes. The combination of quinoa and bell peppers ensures a nutrient-dense meal that is satisfying and nourishing.

The choice between lean ground turkey or tofu provides added flexibility for those following different dietary preferences. Lean ground turkey is a rich source of lean protein, which is vital for muscle building and repair. It is also a low-fat option that can help maintain a healthy weight, which is important for managing prediabetes. On the other hand, tofu is a plant-based protein that is suitable for vegetarians and vegans. It is low in saturated fat and cholesterol, making it heart-healthy and suitable for those with prediabetes.

To prepare this wholesome dish, start by preheating the oven and cooking the quinoa according to package instructions. Meanwhile, prepare the bell peppers by cutting off the tops and removing the seeds. In a pan, cook the ground turkey or tofu with olive oil and seasonings until fully cooked. Once the quinoa and protein are ready, combine them in a mixing bowl and stuff the mixture into the bell peppers. Bake in the oven until the peppers are tender and the filling is golden brown.

In summary, quinoa-stuffed bell peppers with lean ground turkey or tofu is a nutritious and flavorful option for individuals with prediabetes. The combination of quinoa, fiber-packed bell peppers, and a choice between lean protein sources provides a well-rounded meal that supports blood sugar regulation, weight management, and overall health.

SPINACH AND FETA OMELET WITH WHOLE WHEAT TOAST

A spinach and feta omelet with whole wheat toast is a delicious and nutritious option for individuals with prediabetes. Packed with essential nutrients and low in carbohydrates, this dish is a great choice to help regulate blood sugar levels and promote overall health.

Spinach, a leafy green vegetable, is the star ingredient of this omelet. It is rich in vitamins A, C, and K, as well as important minerals like iron and magnesium. Spinach is also low in calories and high in fiber, making it an excellent choice for managing prediabetes. Fiber helps slow down the digestion of carbohydrates, preventing rapid spikes in blood sugar levels.

Adding feta cheese to the omelet not only enhances the flavor but also provides additional nutritional benefits. Feta cheese is a good source of protein, calcium, and vitamins B6 and B12. Protein is important for managing prediabetes as it slows down the absorption of glucose, preventing blood sugar spikes. Calcium helps maintain bone health, while vitamins B6 and B12 support the proper functioning of the nervous system.

The omelet is paired with whole wheat toast, which is a healthier alternative to refined white bread. Whole wheat bread is higher in fiber and contains essential nutrients such as folate, magnesium, and selenium. The high fiber content helps control blood sugar levels and promotes better digestion.

To prepare this nutritious dish, whisk together eggs, a handful of fresh spinach leaves, and crumbled feta cheese in a bowl. Heat a non-stick pan over medium heat and pour the egg mixture into the pan, allowing it to cook for a few minutes until the edges begin to set. Gently fold the omelet in half and let it cook for a couple more minutes until the inside is cooked through. Serve the omelet with a slice of toasted whole wheat bread for a complete and satisfying meal.

In conclusion, a spinach and feta omelet with whole wheat toast is a healthy and delicious option for individuals with prediabetes. Packed with essential nutrients, low in carbohydrates, and high in fiber, this dish helps regulate blood sugar levels and provides numerous health benefits.

BAKED TOFU WITH ROASTED SWEET POTATOES AND STEAMED GREEN BEANS

Baked tofu with roasted sweet potatoes and steamed green beans is a delicious and nutritious meal that is particularly beneficial for individuals with prediabetes. Tofu, made from soybeans, is an excellent plant-based source of protein which helps stabilize blood sugar levels and improve insulin sensitivity. It is also low in fat and cholesterol-free, making it a heart-healthy option for those at risk of developing diabetes. The roasted sweet potatoes provide a satisfying sweetness while also supplying fiber, vitamins, and minerals. The high fiber content in sweet potatoes helps regulate blood sugar levels by slowing down the digestion and absorption of carbohydrates. Furthermore, they are rich in beta-carotene, an antioxidant that may reduce the risk of developing diabetes-related complications. Steamed green beans, on the other hand, offer a burst of green goodness packed with essential nutrients like vitamin C, vitamin K, and folate. These nutrients contribute to improved blood circulation, immune function, and overall health. The combination of the three main ingredients in this dish offers a balanced meal that is low in calories and high in nutrients, making it an ideal choice for individuals with prediabetes who aim to manage their blood sugar levels and maintain a healthy weight.

To prepare this wholesome meal, start by preheating the oven to 400°F (200°C). Cut the tofu into cubes and toss them in a marinade of your choice, such as soy sauce, garlic, and ginger. While the tofu marinates, peel and dice the sweet potatoes into bite-sized pieces. Toss the sweet potatoes in olive oil, salt, and any desired seasoning, such as paprika or cinnamon. Arrange the marinated tofu and seasoned sweet potatoes on a baking sheet and roast in the oven for about 25-30 minutes until they are golden and crispy. Meanwhile, steam the green beans for about 5-7 minutes until they are tender but still bright green. Once everything is cooked, serve the baked tofu on a bed of roasted sweet potatoes, with a side of steamed green beans. This colorful and flavorful dish will not only satisfy your taste buds but also contribute to your overall health and wellbeing if you have prediabetes.

BLACK BEAN AND VEGETABLE ENCHILADAS WITH A SIDE OF SALSA AND BROWN RICE

Black bean and vegetable enchiladas with a side of salsa and brown rice are a delicious and wholesome option for those with prediabetes. This flavorful and nutritious dish is packed with various benefits that can help individuals manage their blood sugar levels and maintain a healthy lifestyle.

Firstly, black beans are a great source of protein, fiber, and complex carbohydrates, making them an ideal choice for individuals with prediabetes. Protein and fiber help slow down digestion and the release of glucose into the bloodstream, preventing surges in blood sugar levels. Additionally, the complex carbohydrates found in black beans are slowly digested, providing a sustained release of energy and preventing rapid spikes in blood sugar.

Furthermore, incorporating a variety of vegetables into the enchiladas adds essential nutrients while keeping the dish low in calories and carbohydrates. Vegetables such as bell peppers, onions, zucchini, and spinach provide an array of vitamins, minerals, and antioxidants that support overall health. These colorful additions also increase the fiber content of the meal, aiding digestion and promoting a feeling of fullness, which can help individuals maintain a healthy weight and manage blood sugar levels.

To prepare this dish, start by sautéing the vegetables with a touch of olive oil until they become tender. Then, mix in the black beans and season with spices like cumin, paprika, and chili powder for added flavor. Once the filling is ready, carefully spoon it onto corn tortillas, roll them up, and place them in a baking dish. Top the enchiladas with a homemade salsa made from diced tomatoes, onions, cilantro, lime juice, and a touch of jalapeno for a zesty kick. Bake the enchiladas until the tortillas are crispy and the flavors are melded together. Serve the enchiladas alongside a portion of nutty brown rice for a well-rounded and satisfying meal.

In conclusion, black bean and vegetable enchiladas with a side of salsa and brown rice provide a wholesome and diabetes-friendly option for individuals managing prediabetes. The combination of protein, fiber, and complex carbohydrates in black beans, along with the nutrient-rich vegetables and low glycemic index of brown rice, can help individuals maintain stable blood sugar levels while enjoying a delicious and satisfying meal.

GRILLED SHRIMP SKEWERS WITH A SIDE SALAD AND WHOLE GRAIN COUSCOUS

Grilled shrimp skewers with a side salad and whole grain couscous is a delicious and healthy meal that offers numerous benefits for individuals with prediabetes. Shrimp is a low-calorie, lean source of protein that is rich in omega-3 fatty acids, which have been shown to improve insulin sensitivity and reduce inflammation in the body. Additionally, shrimp contains essential vitamins and minerals like vitamin B12, selenium, and zinc, which support cardiovascular health and aid in the regulation of blood sugar levels.

Pairing the grilled shrimp skewers with a side salad and whole grain couscous adds even more nutritional value to the meal. The side salad provides an abundance of fiber and various vegetables, such as leafy greens, tomatoes, cucumbers, and bell peppers, which are all low in calories but high in vitamins, minerals, and antioxidants. The combination of fiber and antioxidants assists in managing blood sugar levels, promoting satiety, and preventing the development of more severe conditions associated with prediabetes.

Incorporating whole grain couscous into the dish

not only enhances its taste and texture but also contributes to its health benefits. Whole grain couscous is an excellent source of complex carbohydrates, fiber, and essential nutrients like magnesium and phosphorus. These nutrients help slow down the digestion process and prevent sudden spikes in blood sugar levels. Furthermore, the high fiber content aids in weight management by promoting a feeling of fullness and reducing the overall caloric intake.

VEGGIE AND BEAN BURRITO BOWL WITH BROWN RICE AND SALSA

Veggie and bean burrito bowl with brown rice and salsa is a delicious and nutritious option for individuals with prediabetes. This hearty meal is packed with numerous benefits that can help manage blood sugar levels and promote overall health.

Starting with the brown rice, it is a complex carbohydrate that is low on the glycemic index, meaning it has a slower and steadier impact on blood sugar levels compared to white rice. Brown rice is also a good source of fiber, which aids in digestion and helps control blood sugar. It is rich in essential nutrients such as magnesium and B vitamins, which are beneficial for individuals with prediabetes.

Additionally, the veggie and bean components of this burrito bowl provide a wide array of nutrients without the added sugars and refined carbs commonly found in other dishes. Vegetables like bell peppers, onions, and tomatoes are packed with vitamins and minerals, as well as fiber. Beans, such as black beans or pinto beans, are an excellent source of plant-based protein and fiber that help regulate blood sugar levels.

To prepare this flavorful bowl, start by cooking the brown rice according to package instructions. While the rice is cooking, sauté a mixture of bell peppers, onions, and any other desired vegetables in a little olive oil until tender. Add in the beans and warm them through. You can season the mixture with spices like cumin, paprika, and chili powder for extra flavor.

Once the rice and vegetables are ready, assemble your burrito bowl by placing a generous portion of brown rice as the base. Top it with the sautéed vegetables and beans mixture. You can then add a dollop of salsa or a homemade tomato-based salsa for added zing and freshness. If desired, you can also garnish the bowl with fresh cilantro, avocado slices, or a squeeze of lime.

This veggie and bean burrito bowl with brown rice and salsa not only provides a satisfying and delicious meal option for individuals with prediabetes, but it also helps control blood sugar levels due to its low-glycemic index ingredients. The combination of whole grains, vegetables, and legumes ensures a well-balanced, nutrient-rich dish that is both diabetes-friendly and incredibly tasty.

To prepare this meal, start by marinating the shrimp in a mixture of olive oil, lemon juice, garlic, and herbs. While the shrimp marinates for 20-30 minutes, prepare a side salad by combining mixed greens, cherry tomatoes, cucumber slices, and bell peppers in a bowl. For the whole grain couscous, follow the package instructions and cook it to perfection. Once the shrimp is marinated, thread them onto skewers and grill them for a few minutes on each side until they turn pink and opaque. Serve the grilled shrimp skewers alongside the side salad and whole grain couscous for a wholesome and satisfying meal that supports stable blood sugar levels and good overall health.

HERE IS A COMPREHENSIVE PRE-DIABETIC 2-WEEK MEAL PLAN:

WEEK 1:

Day 1:

Breakfast: Spinach and feta omelet with whole wheat toast

Lunch: Greek salad with grilled chicken

Dinner: Grilled steak with a side salad and roasted sweet potatoes

Day 2:

Breakfast: Quinoa-stuffed bell peppers with lean ground turkey or tofu

Lunch: Turkey chili with mixed beans and vegetables

Dinner: Baked salmon with quinoa and roasted Brussels sprouts

Day 3:

Breakfast: Baked tofu with roasted sweet potatoes and steamed green beans

Lunch: Lemon garlic shrimp with whole wheat pasta and steamed broccoli

Dinner: Grilled chicken breast with steamed vegetables

Day 4:

Breakfast: Quinoa salad with mixed vegetables and grilled shrimp

Lunch: Vegetable stir-fry with tofu or lean beef

Dinner: Baked chicken with brown rice and roasted asparagus

Day 5:

Breakfast: Oatmeal with berries and a sprinkle of nuts

Lunch: Lentil soup with a side of whole grain bread

Dinner: Grilled vegetable wrap with hummus and avocado

Day 6:

Breakfast: Yogurt with mixed berries and a sprinkle of chia seeds

Lunch: Tuna salad on whole grain bread with a side of raw veggies

Dinner: Greek salad with grilled chicken or shrimp

Day 7:

Breakfast: Veggie and bean burrito bowl with brown rice and salsa

Lunch: Black bean and vegetable enchiladas with a side of salsa and brown rice

Dinner: Baked cod with quinoa and sautéed spinach

WEEK 2:

Day 8:

Breakfast: Scrambled eggs with sautéed mushrooms and whole wheat toast

Lunch: Chicken and vegetable curry with cauliflower rice

Dinner: Grilled shrimp skewers with a side salad and whole grain couscous

Day 9:

Breakfast: Quinoa porridge with almond milk, cinnamon, and a sprinkle of berries

Lunch: Baked tofu with quinoa and steamed vegetables

Dinner: Grilled chicken breast with roasted Brussels sprouts and brown rice

Day 10:

Breakfast: Greek yogurt with sliced almonds and a drizzle of honey

Lunch: Hummus and veggie wrap with a side of raw veggies

Dinner: Turkey chili with mixed beans and vegetables

Day 11:

Breakfast: Green smoothie with kale, spinach, banana, and almond milk

Lunch: Lentil and vegetable salad with a side of whole grain bread

Dinner: Baked salmon with quinoa and steamed broccoli

Day 12:

Breakfast: Whole grain toast with avocado and tomato slices

Lunch: Vegetable stir-fry with tofu or lean beef

Dinner: Grilled steak with a side salad and roasted sweet potatoes

Day 13:

Breakfast: Quinoa salad with mixed vegetables and grilled shrimp

Lunch: Lemon garlic shrimp with whole wheat

pasta and steamed broccoli

Dinner: Baked chicken with brown rice and roasted asparagus

Day 14:

Breakfast: Vegetable omelet with a side of whole wheat toast

Lunch: Spinach and feta salad with grilled chicken or shrimp

Dinner: Quinoa-stuffed bell peppers with lean ground turkey or tofu